I0788319

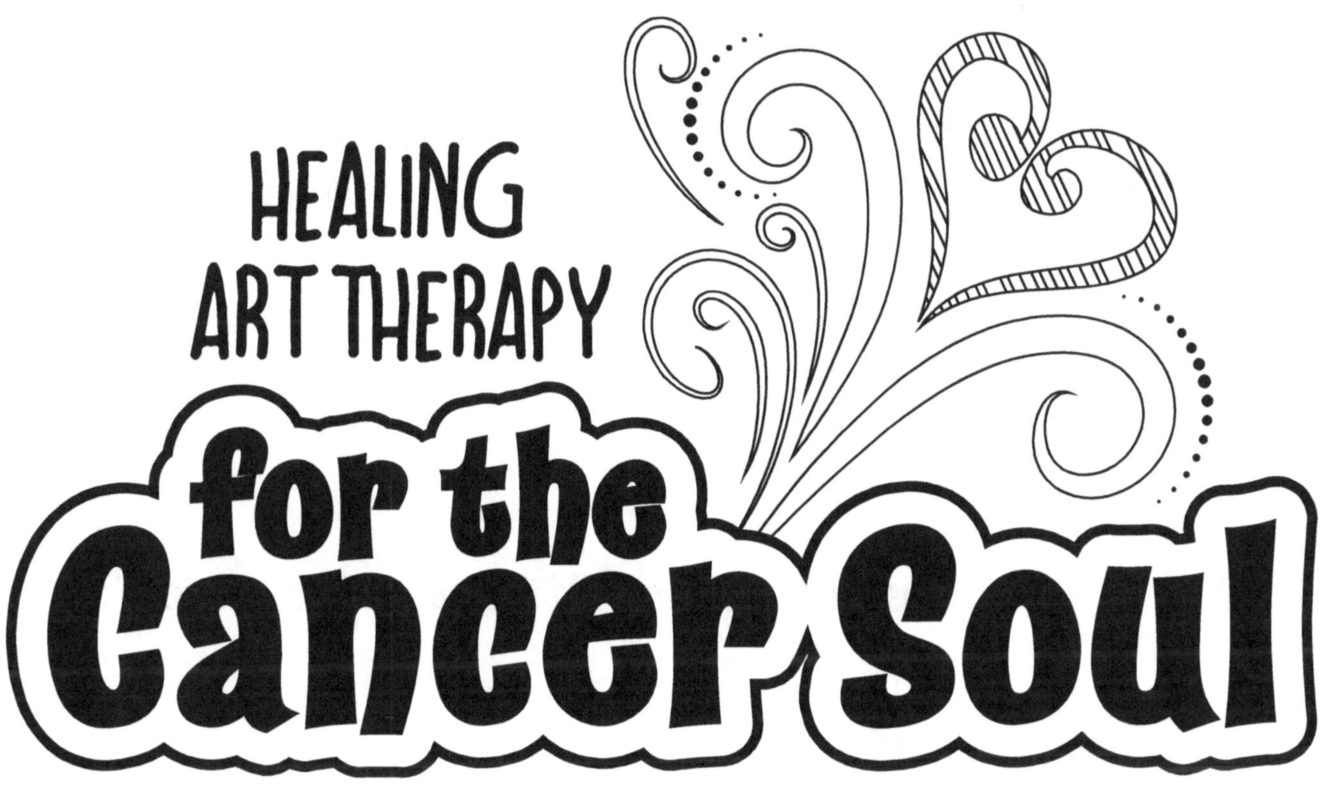

HEALING ART THERAPY for the Cancer Soul

by Marcia McGee Ashford & Roslen Roy Mack

Illustrated by Roslen Roy Mack

Copyright 2020 © Heartstring Productions, LLC., Copyright 2020 © Roslen Roy Mack

All rights reserved. No part of this publication may be reproduced, distributed, or transmitted in any form or by any means, including photocopying, recording, or other electronic or mechanical methods, without the prior written permission of the copyright holders, except in the case of brief quotations, embodied in critical reviews and certain other noncommercial uses permitted by copyright law.

Dedicated to all the Angels in my life; Amber, Alex, Beverly, Matt, Samantha, Mike, Lynn, Chris, Lynn A, Amelia, Jamie, Janice, Mary Drake and Lexi Grace. **-Marcia Ashford**

To Alex and Sam, you are the little blessings that influence my every dream. To Doug, thank you for always being my rock. **-Roslen Mack**

Dedicated to those on their own cancer journey and their support team. You got this!

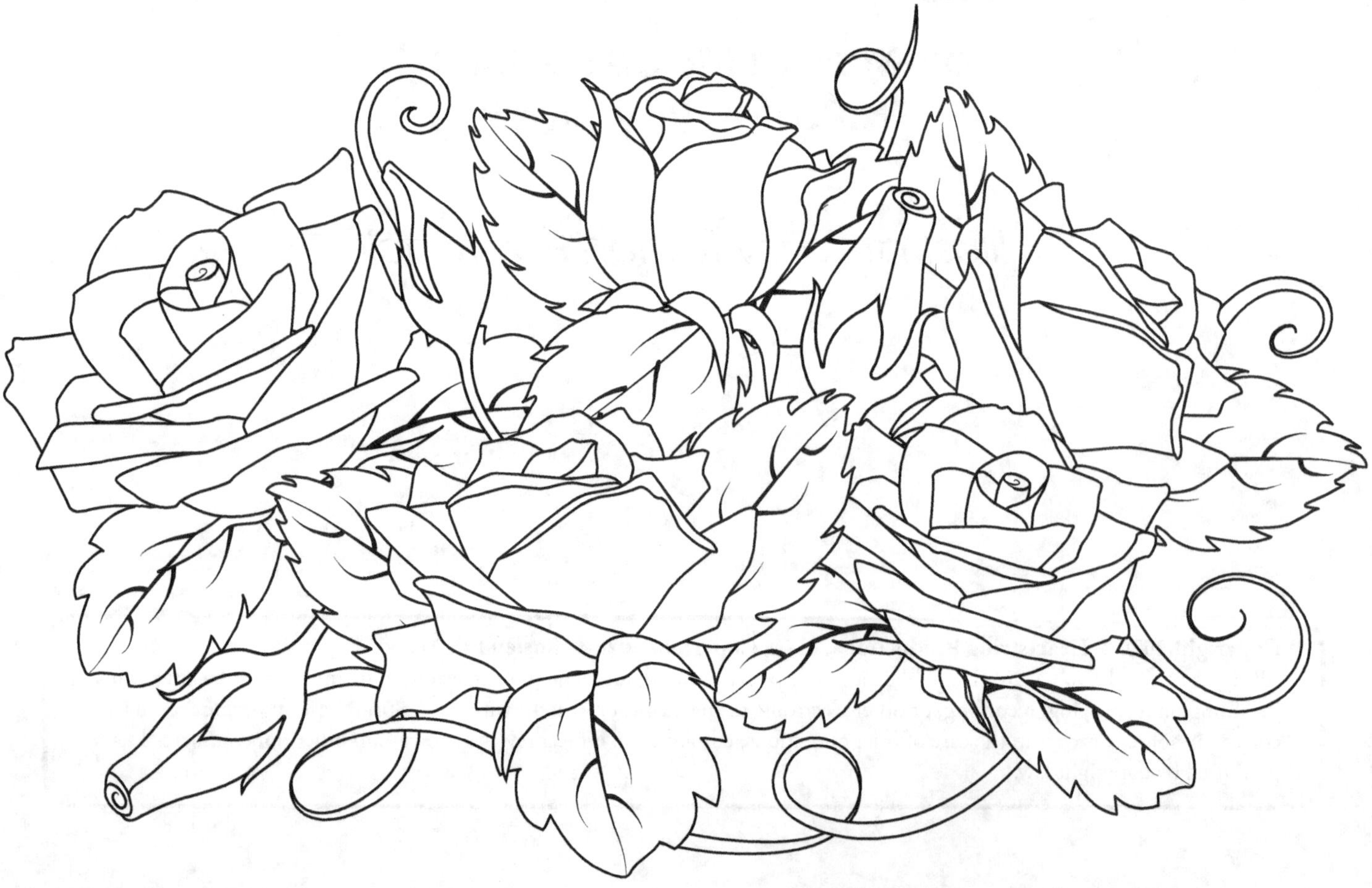

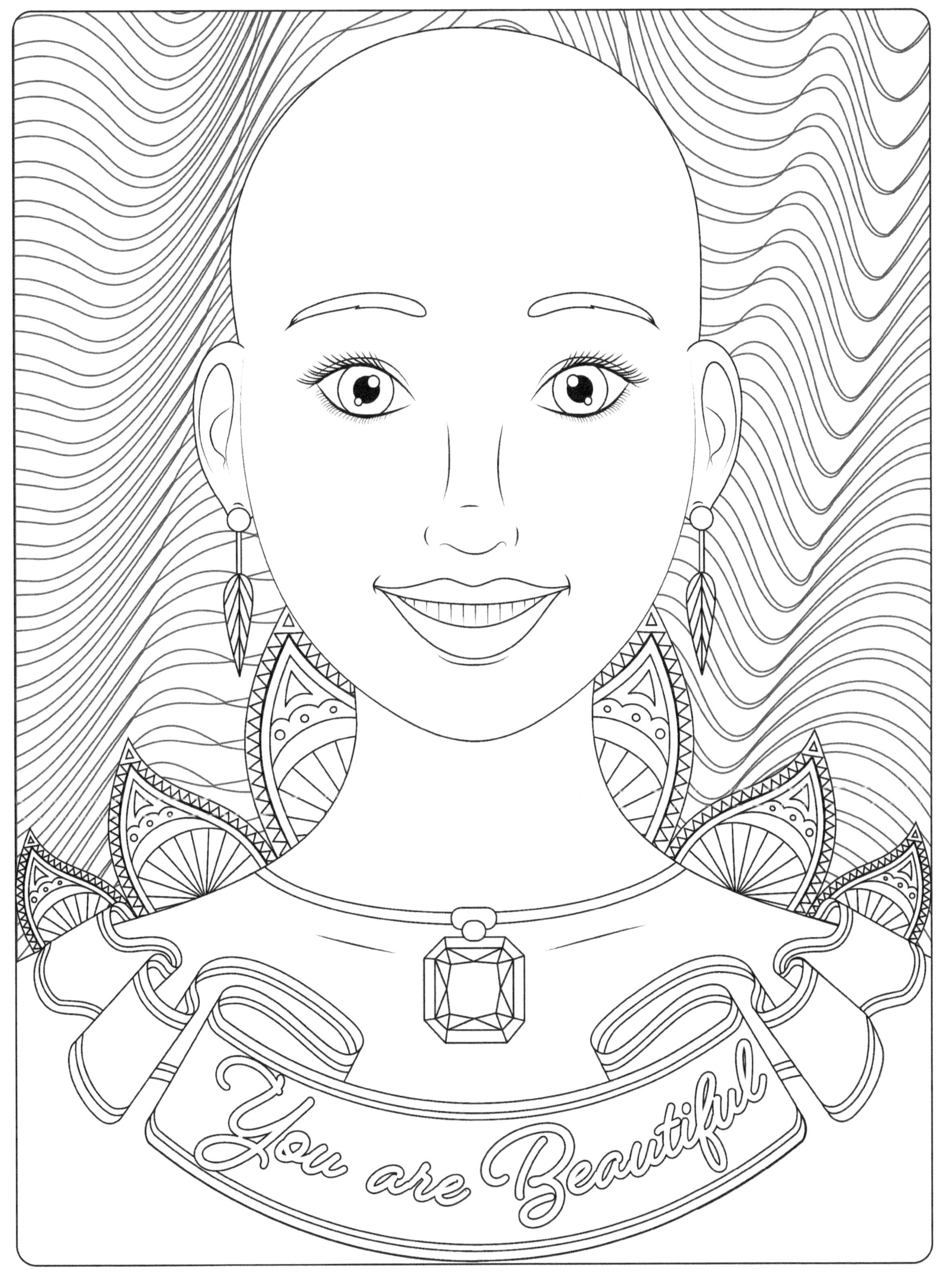
You are Beautiful

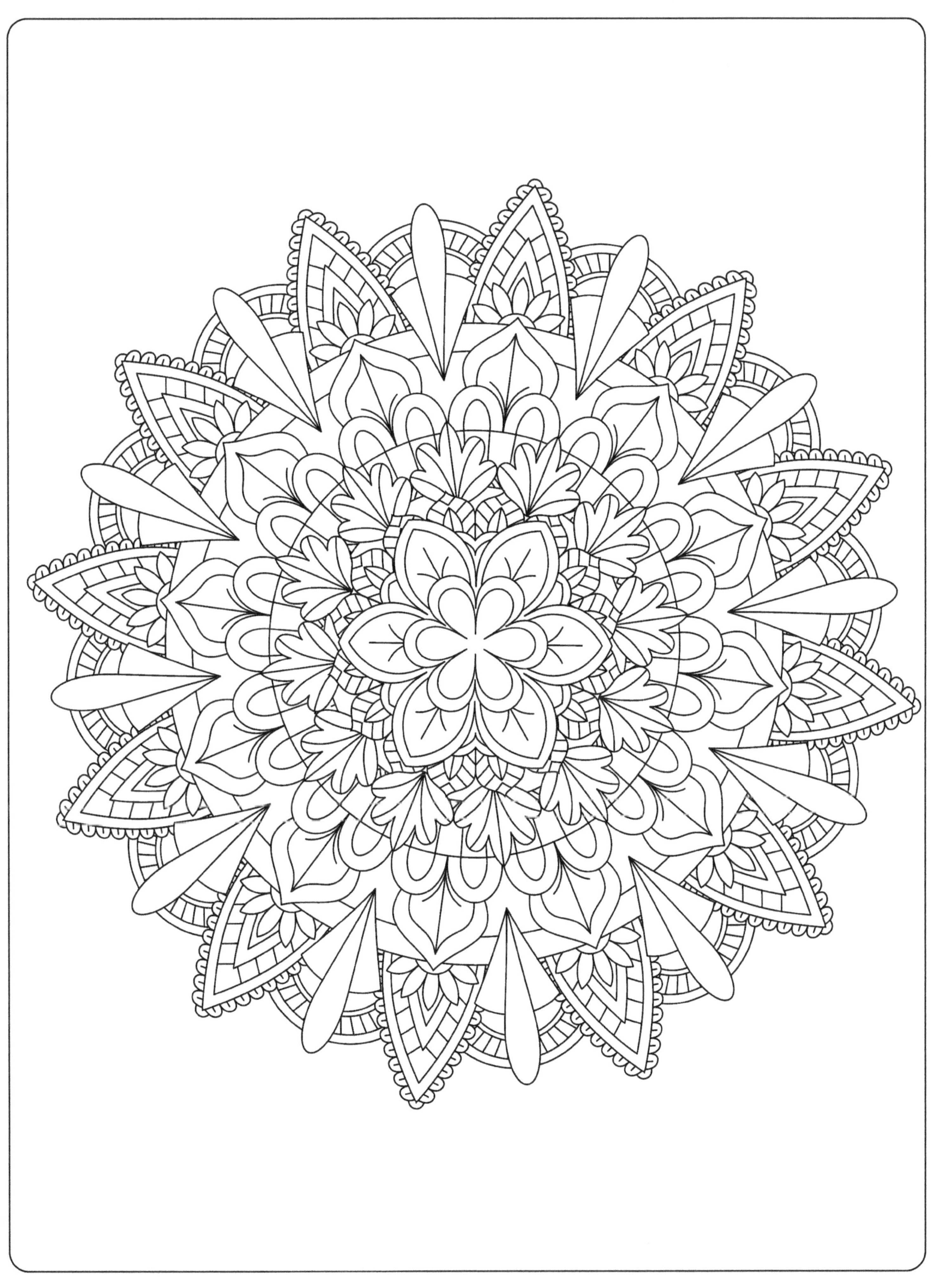

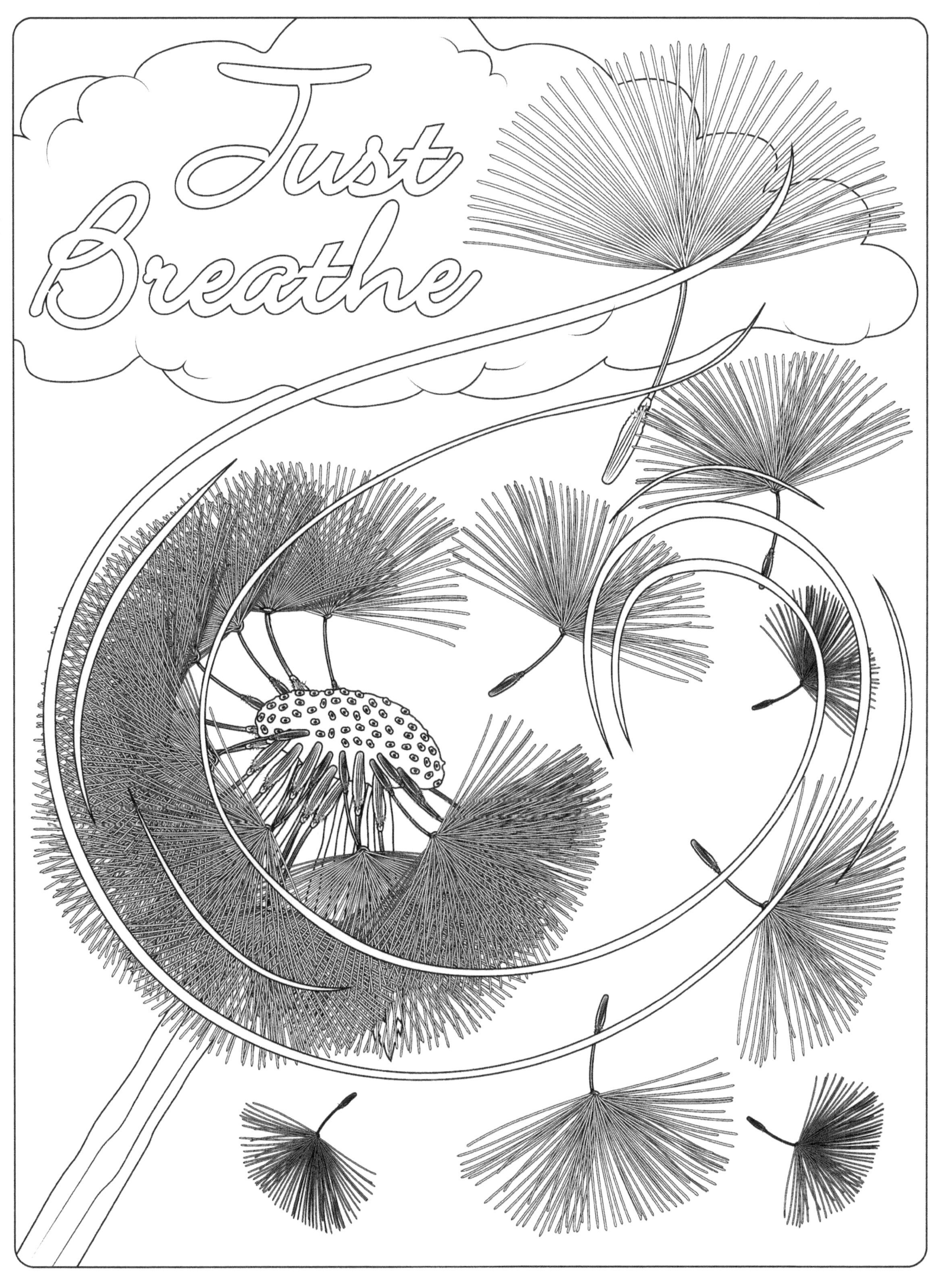

Just
Breathe

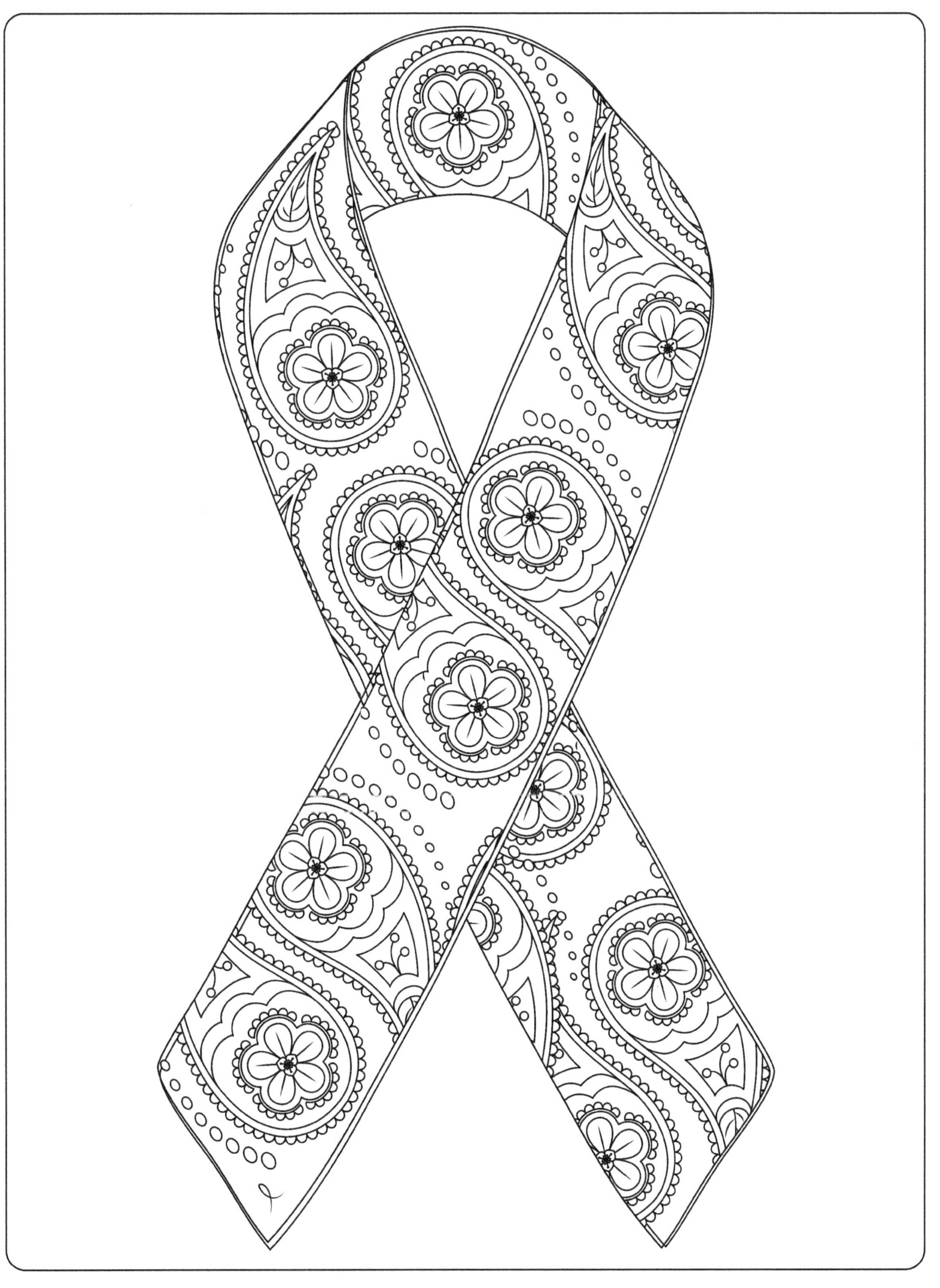

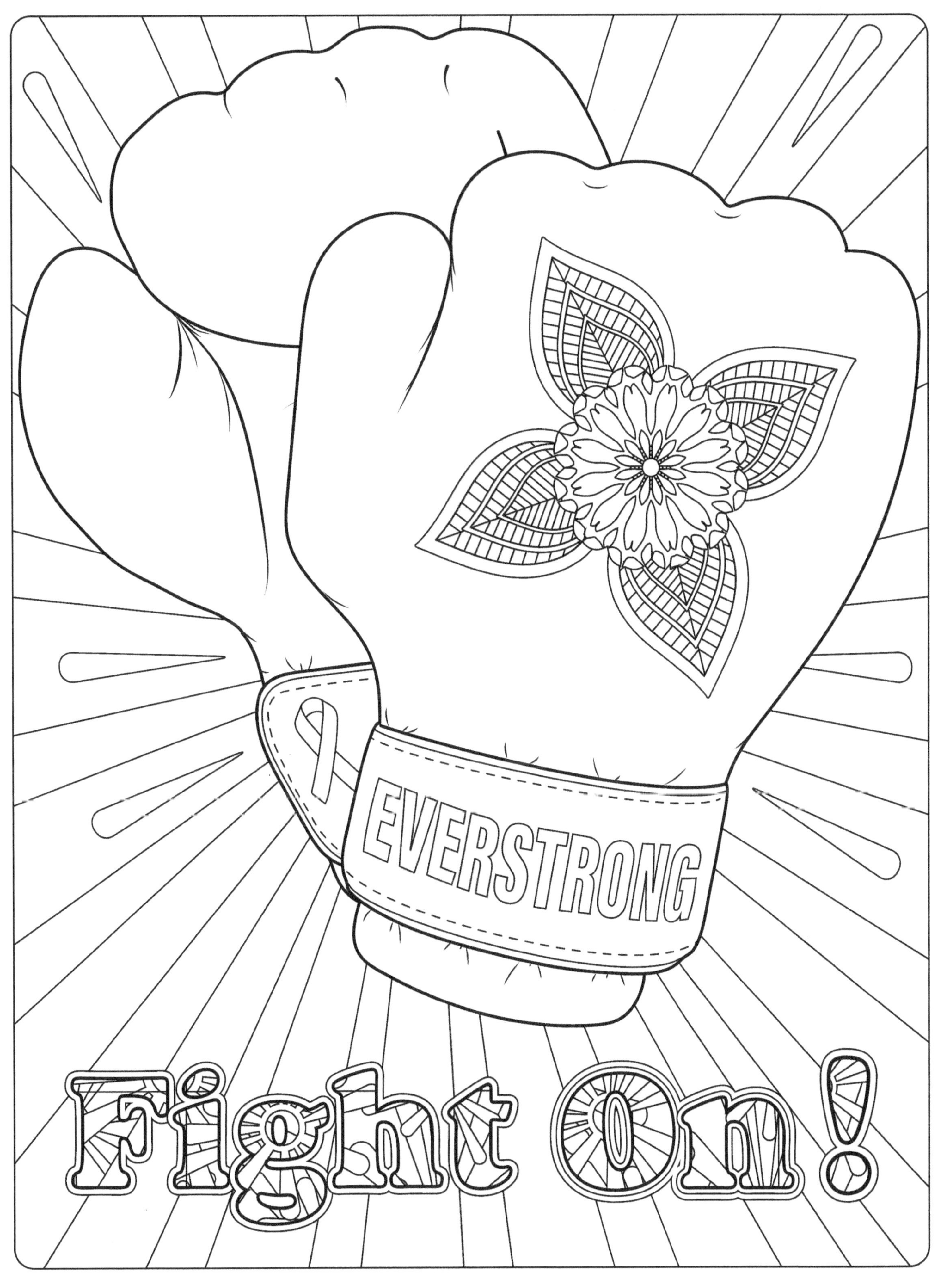

EVERSTRONG
Fight On!

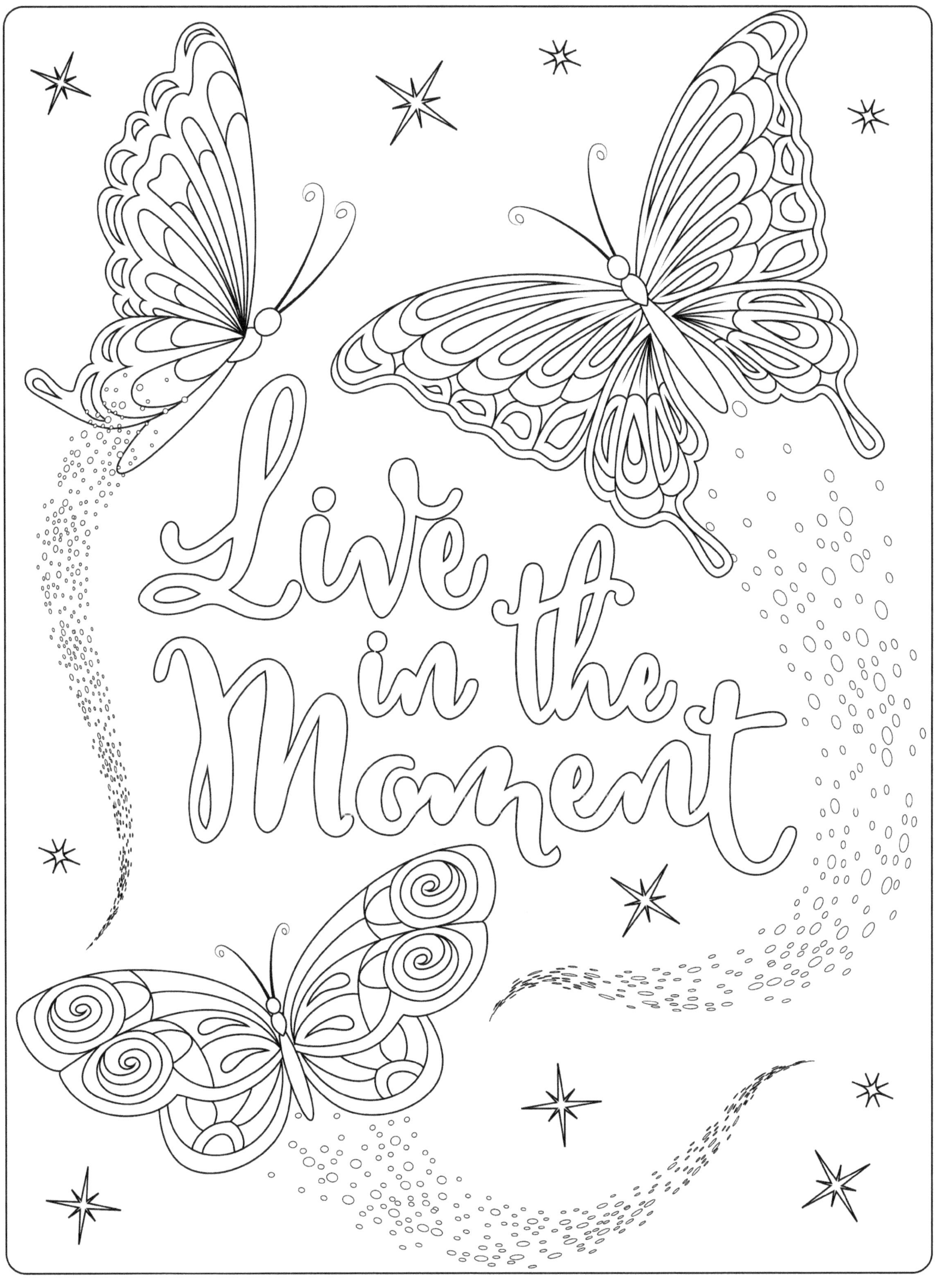

Live in the
Moment

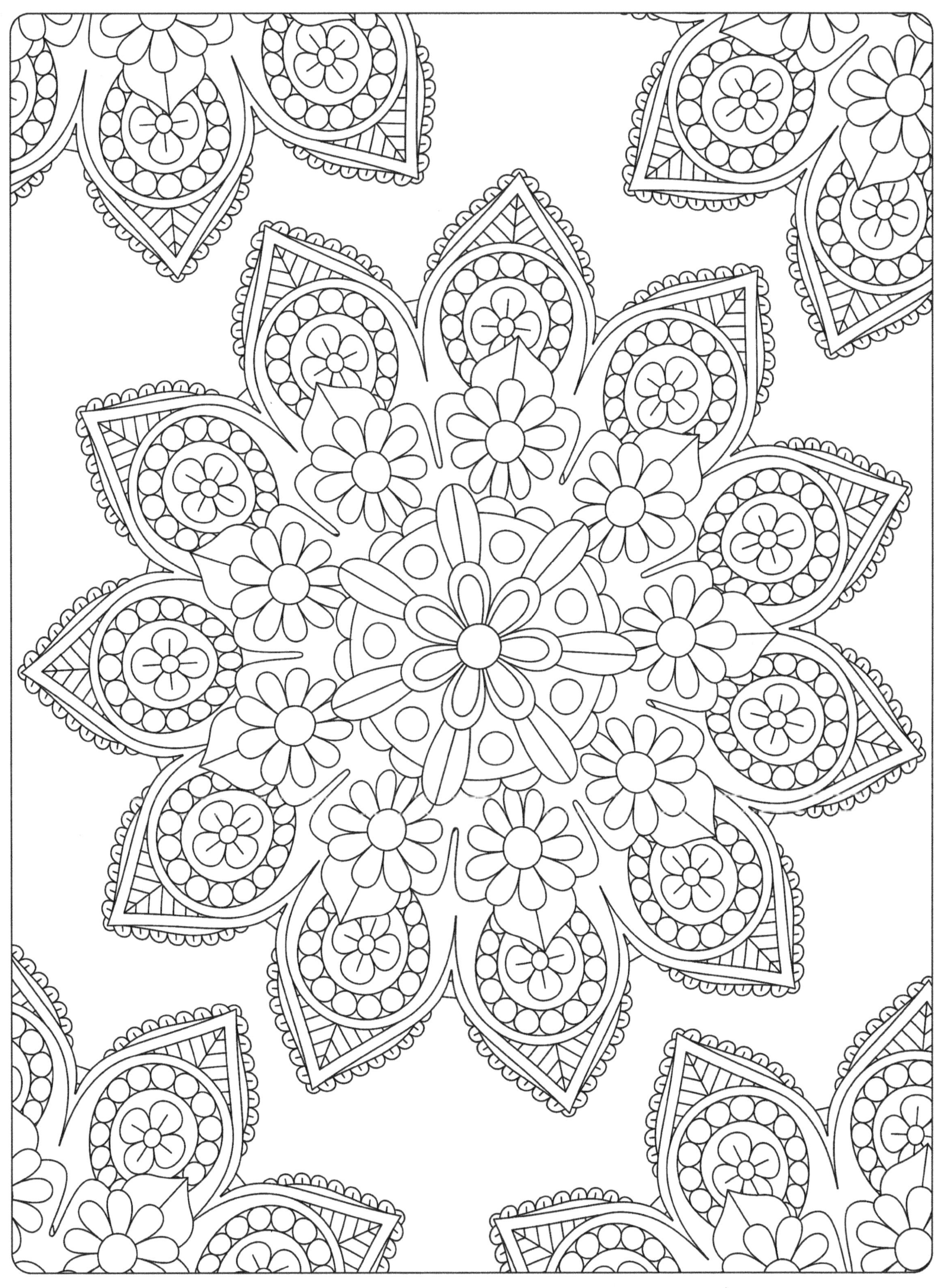

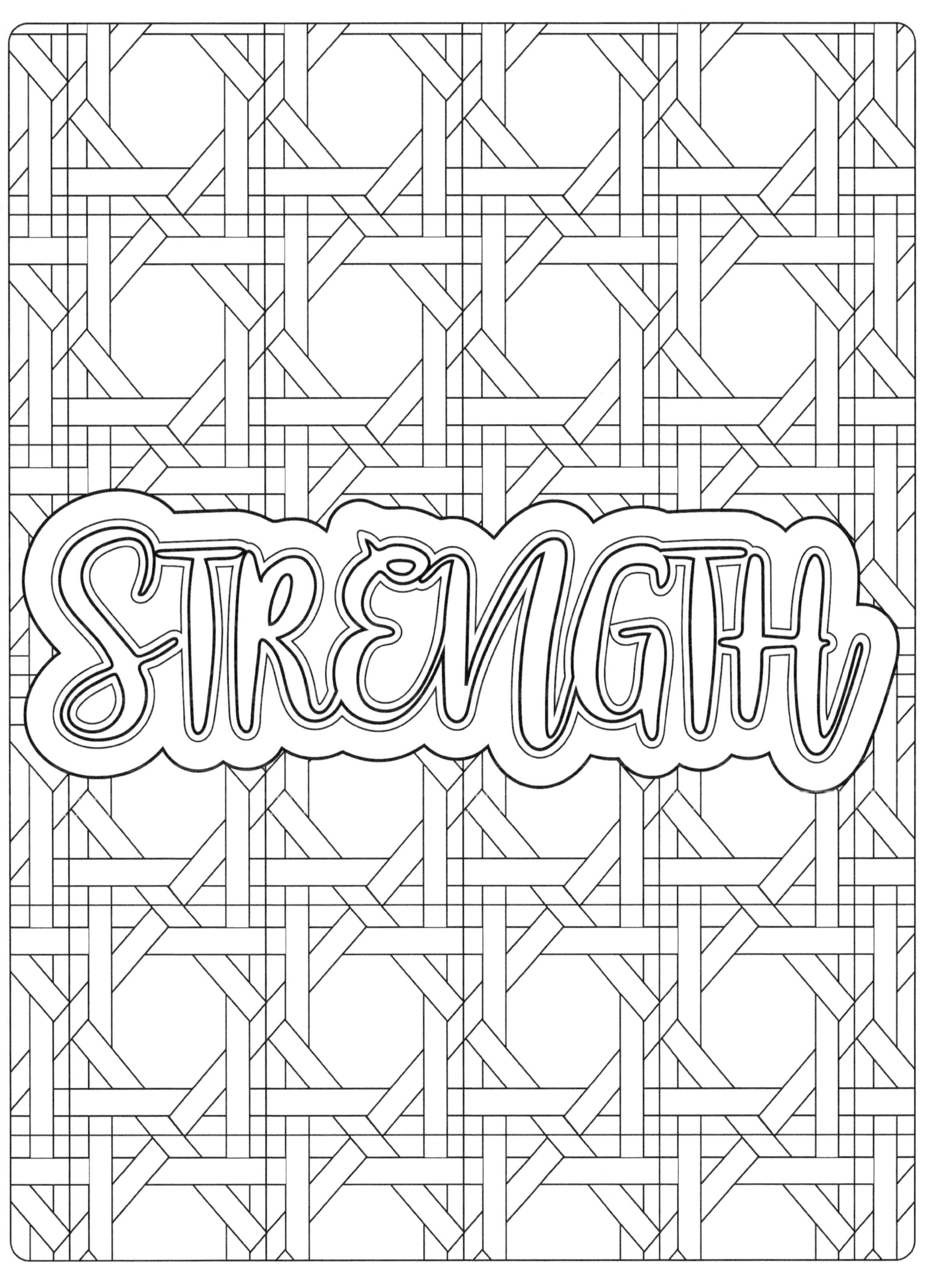
STRENGTH

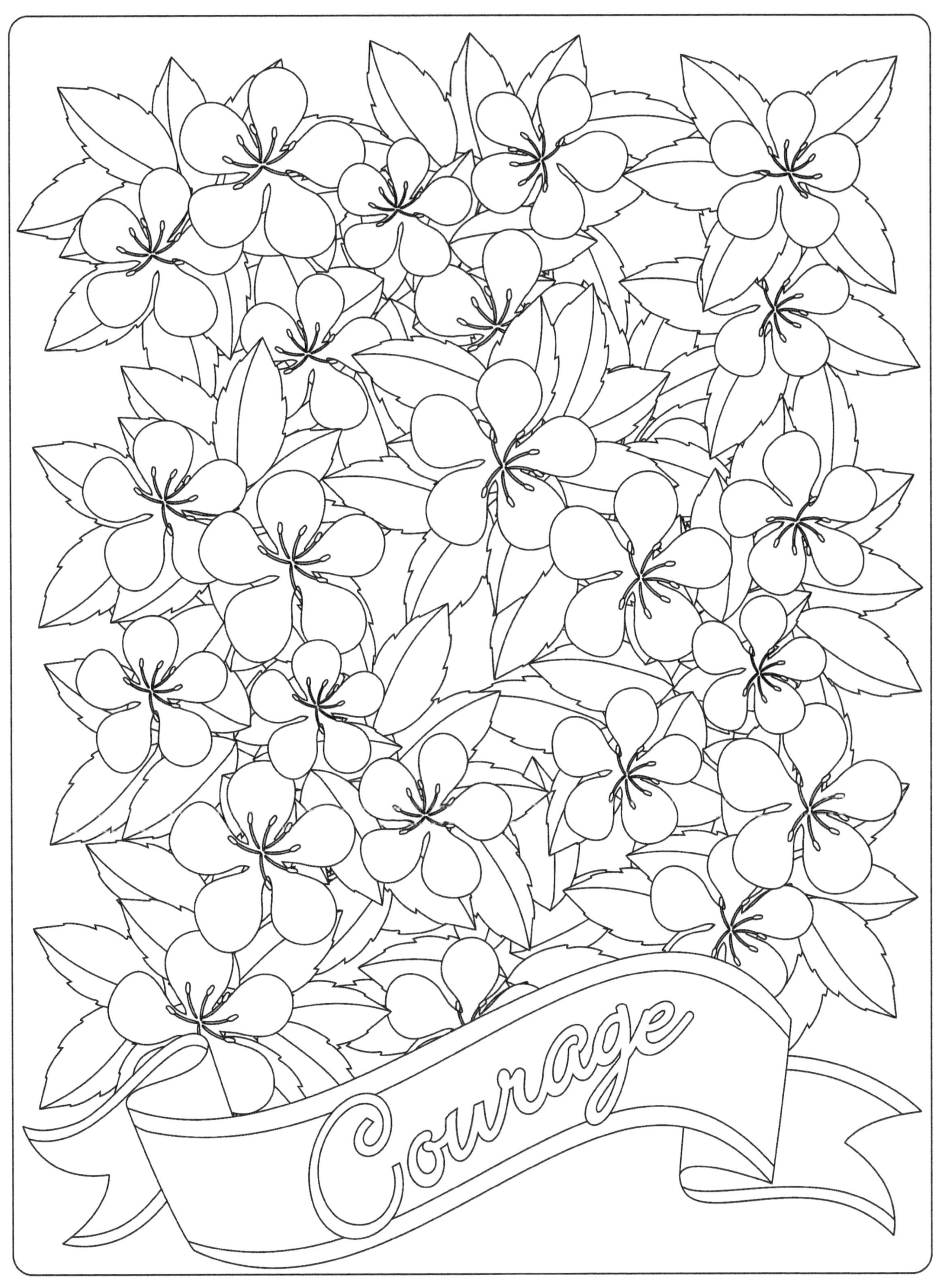

Courage

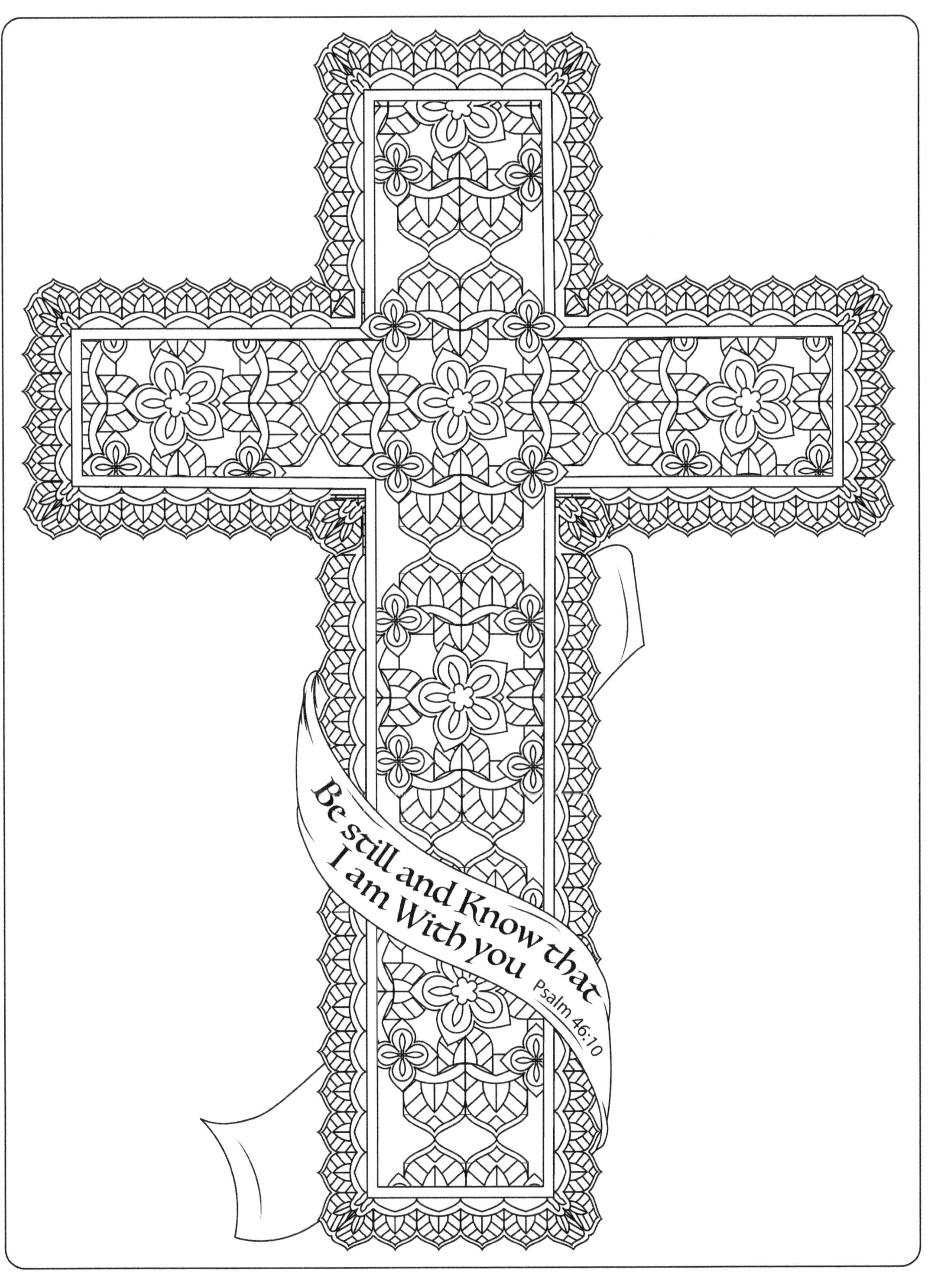

Be still and Know that
I am With you   Psalm 46:10

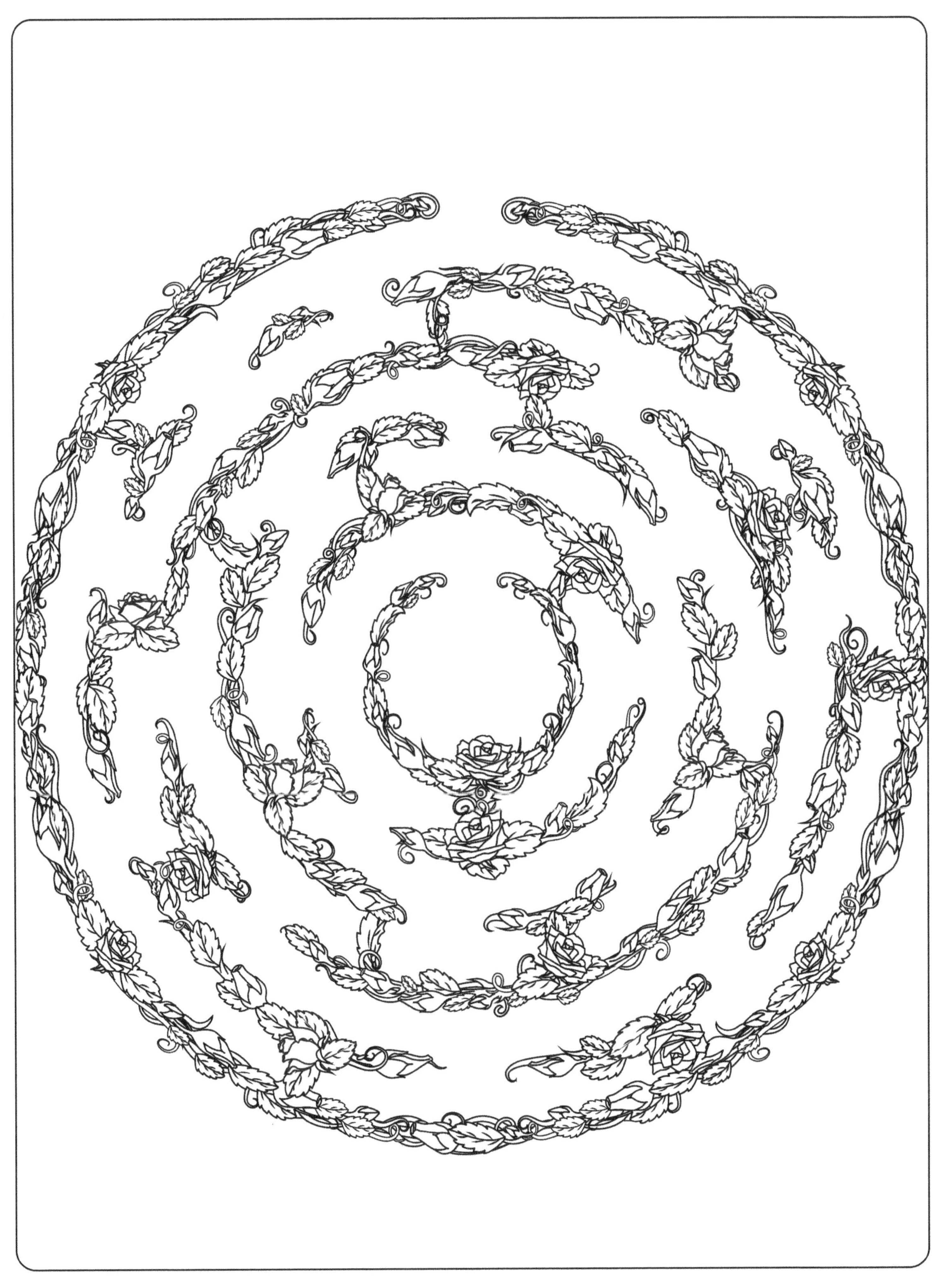

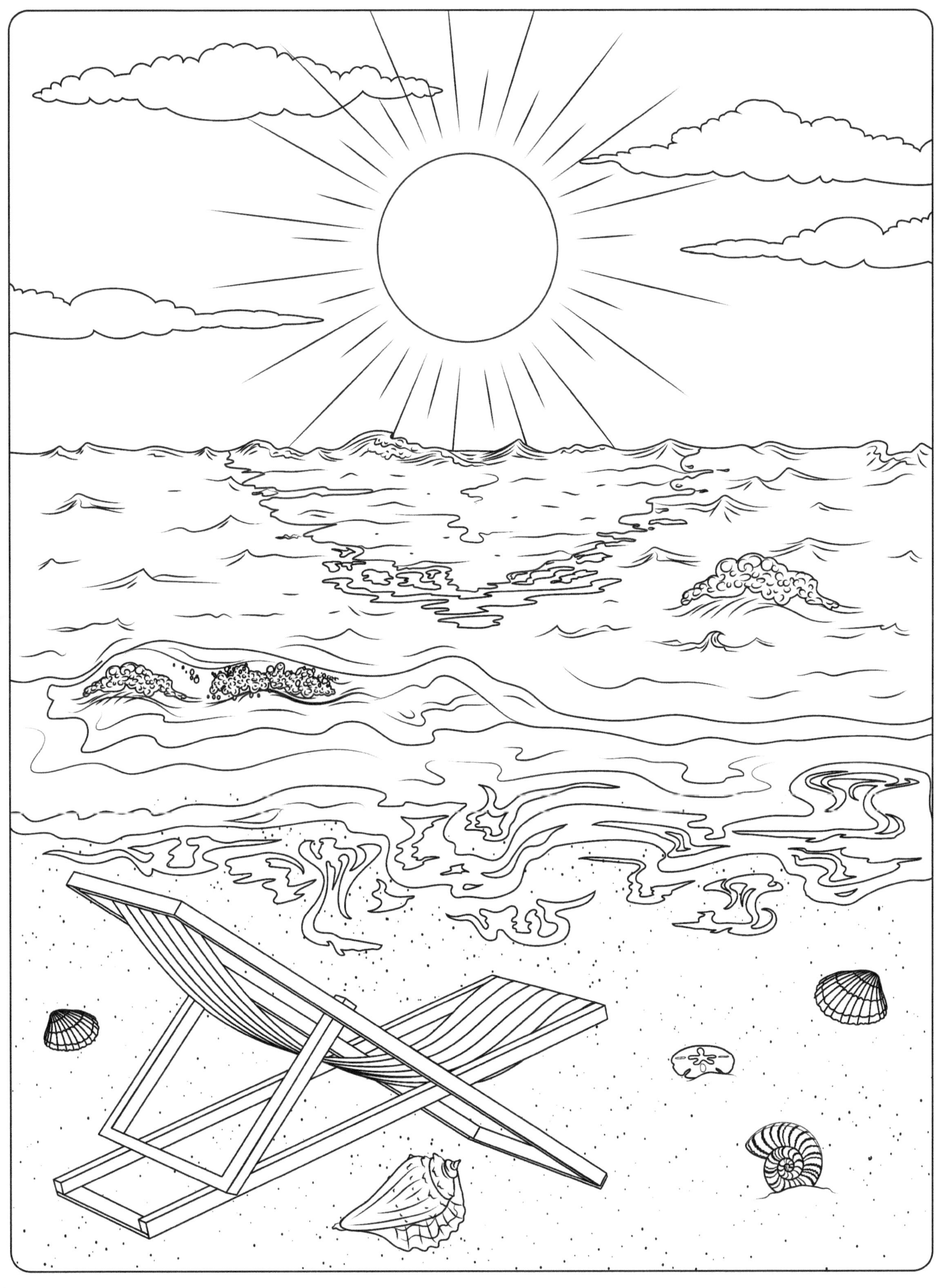

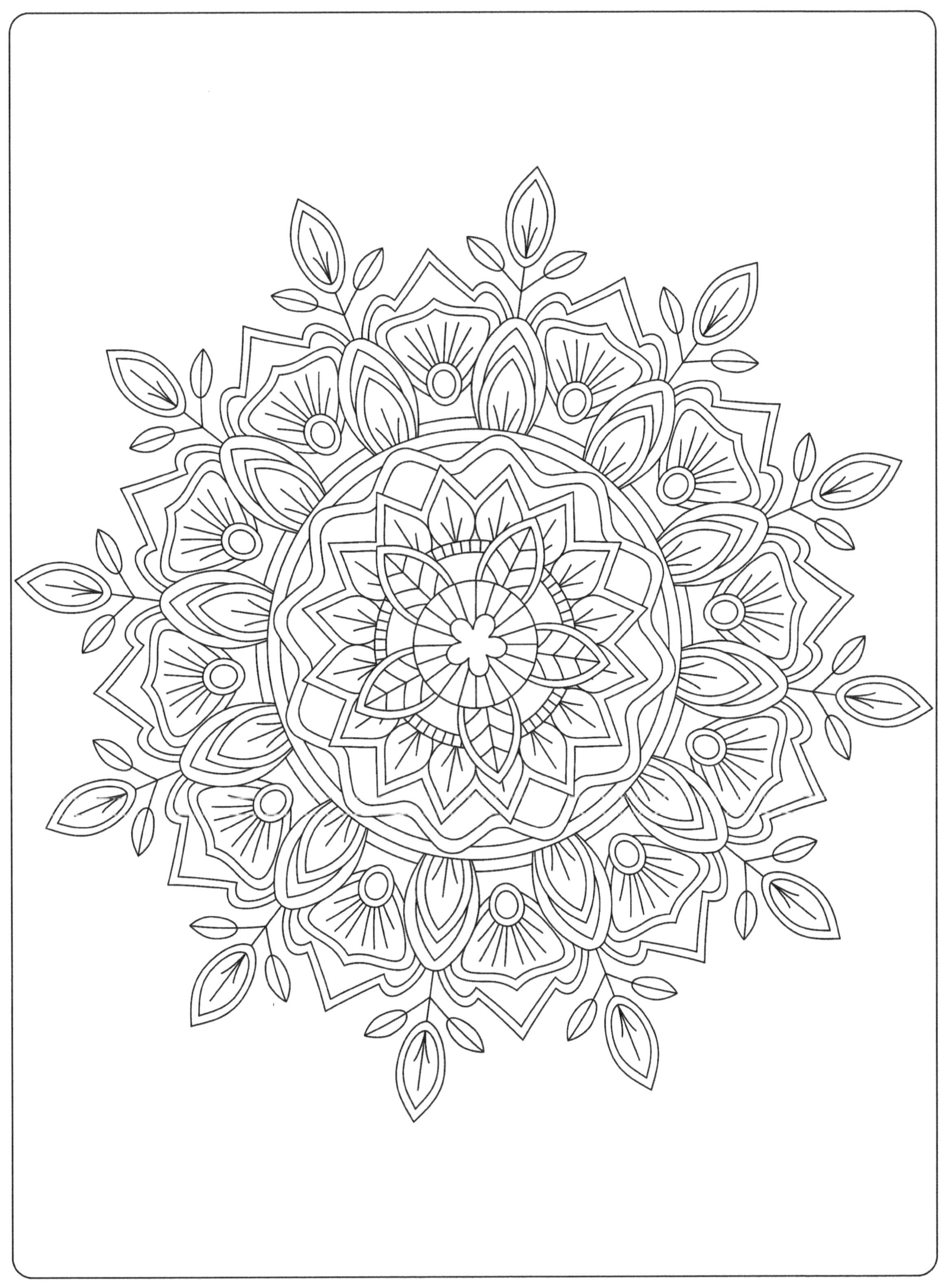

Love

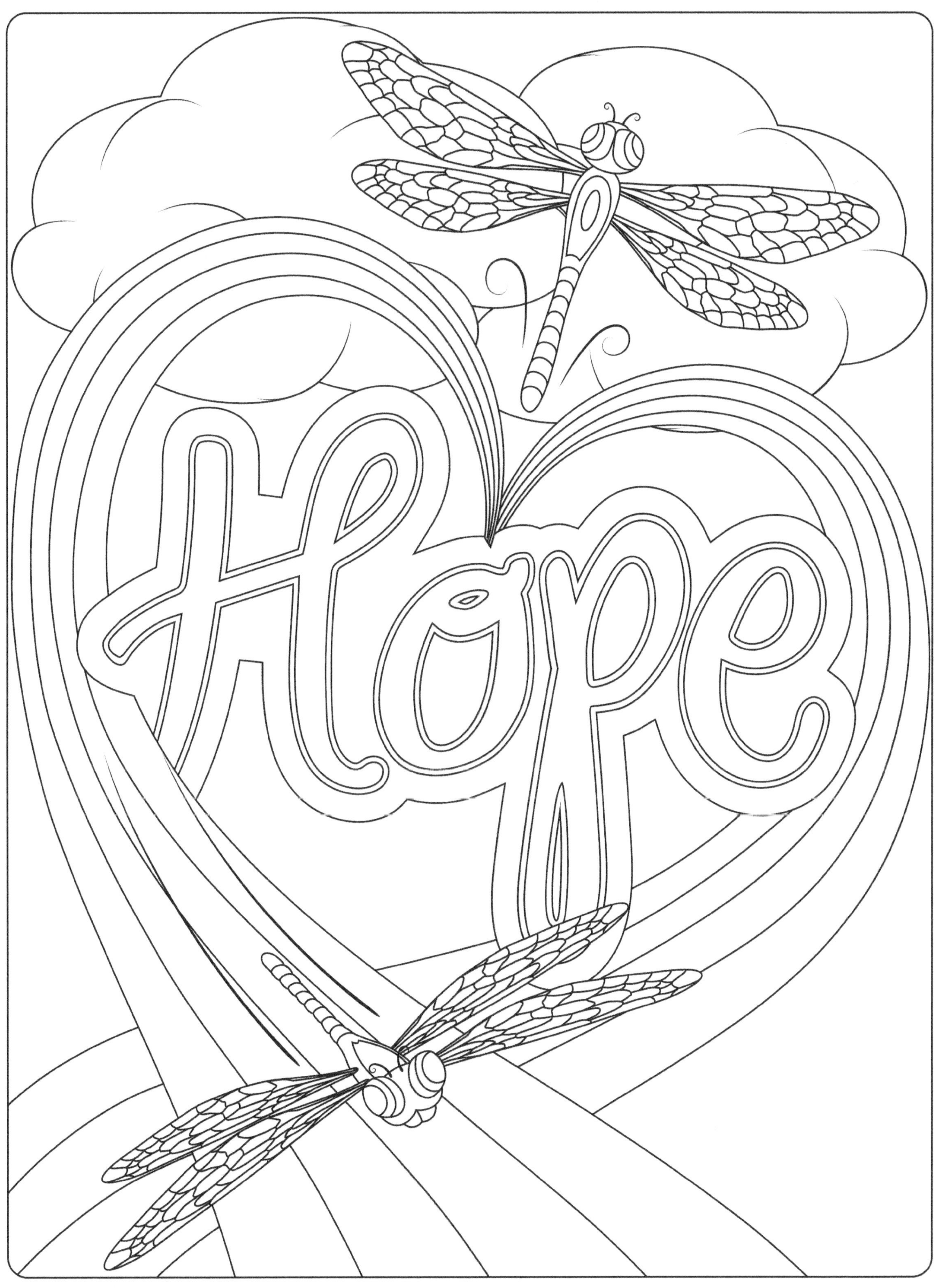
Hope

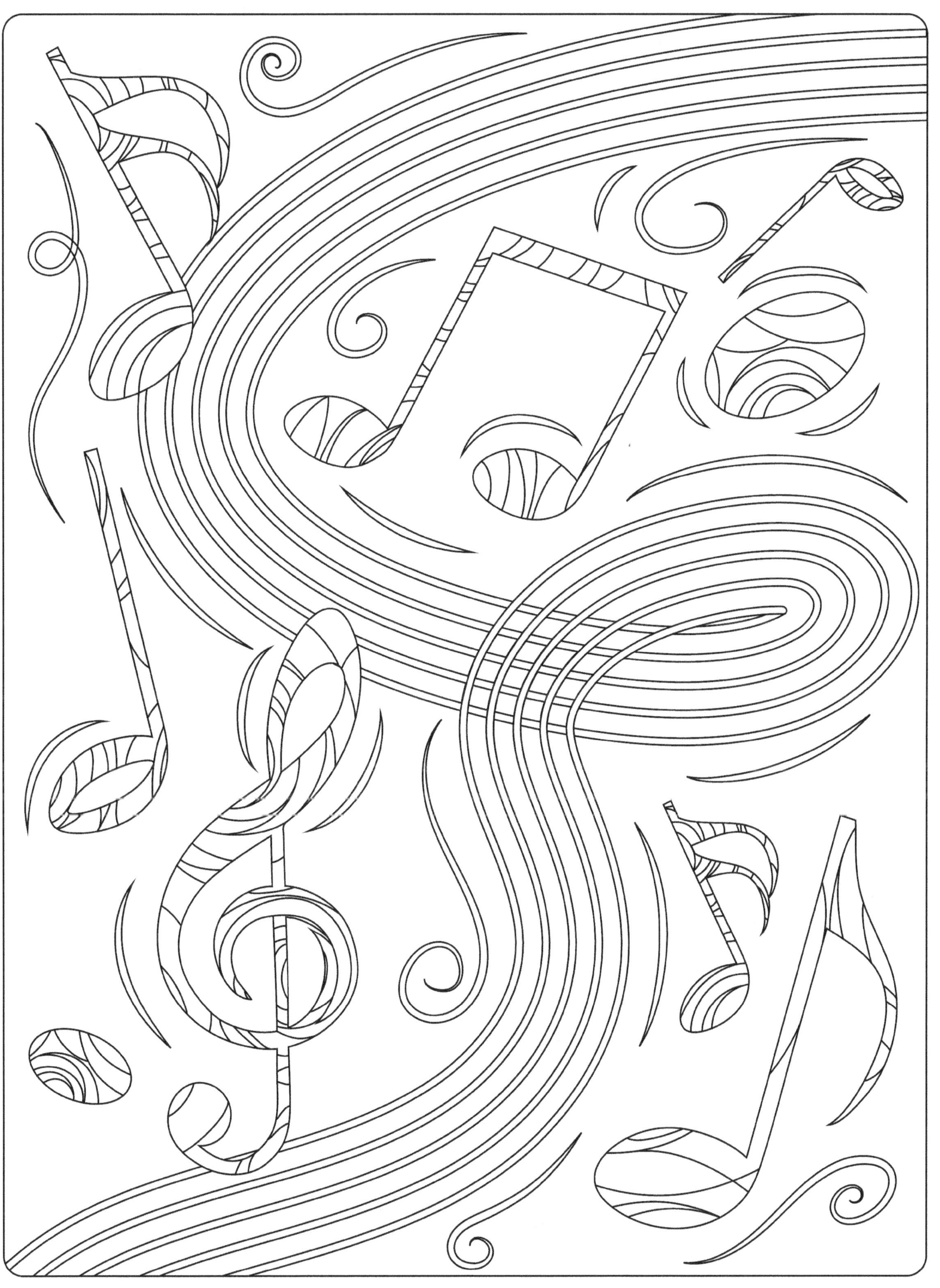

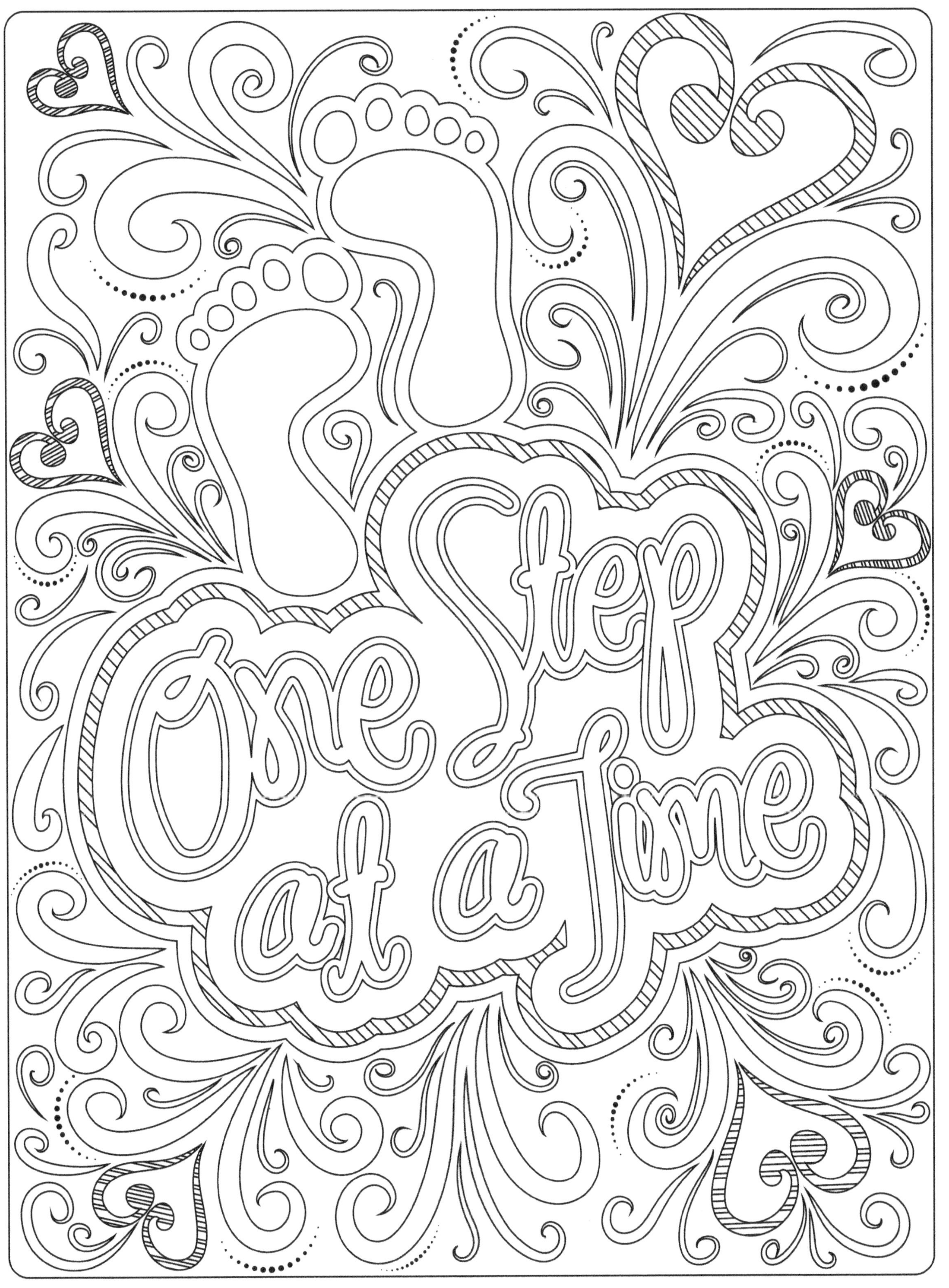

One step
at a time

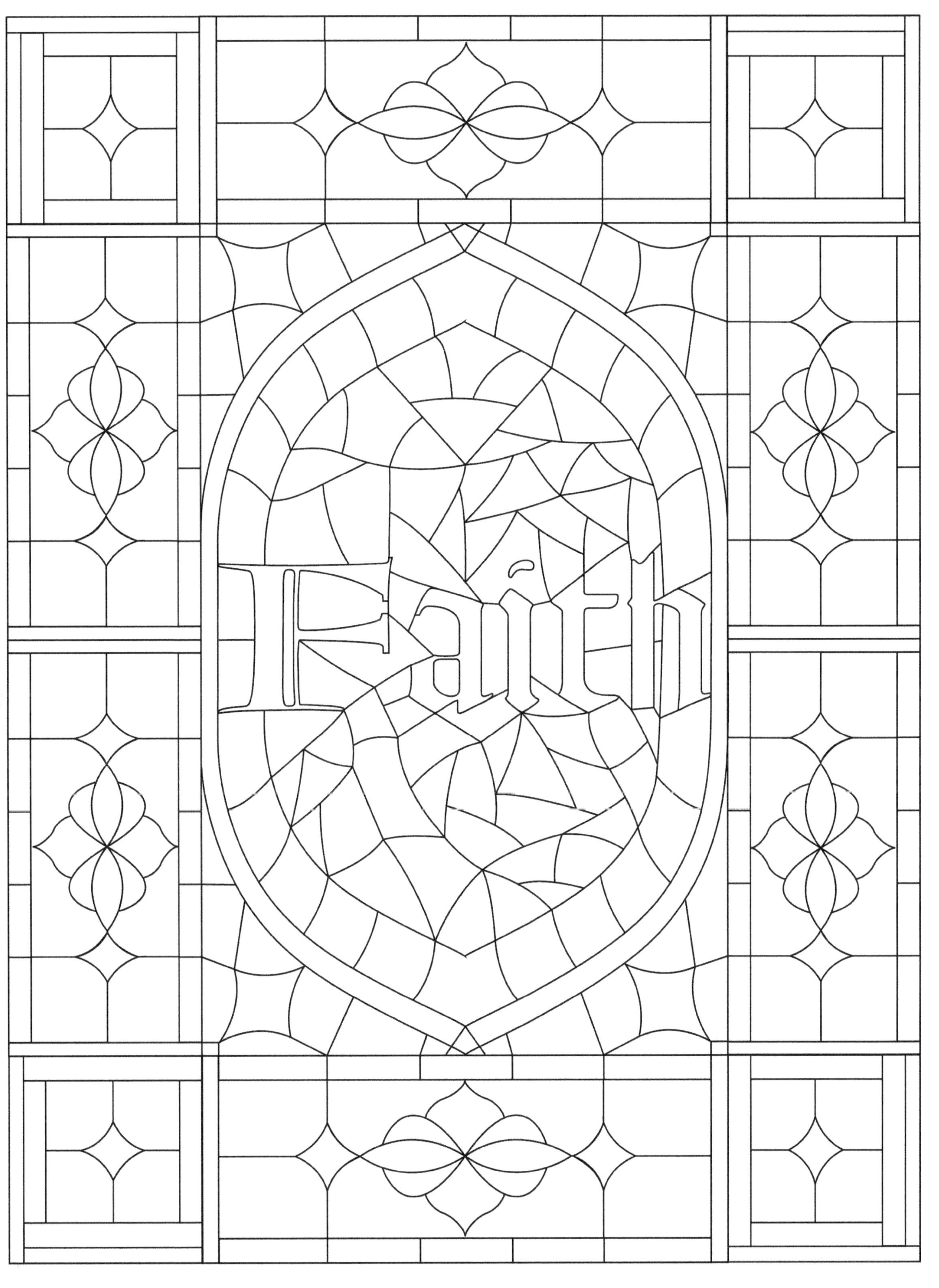
Faith

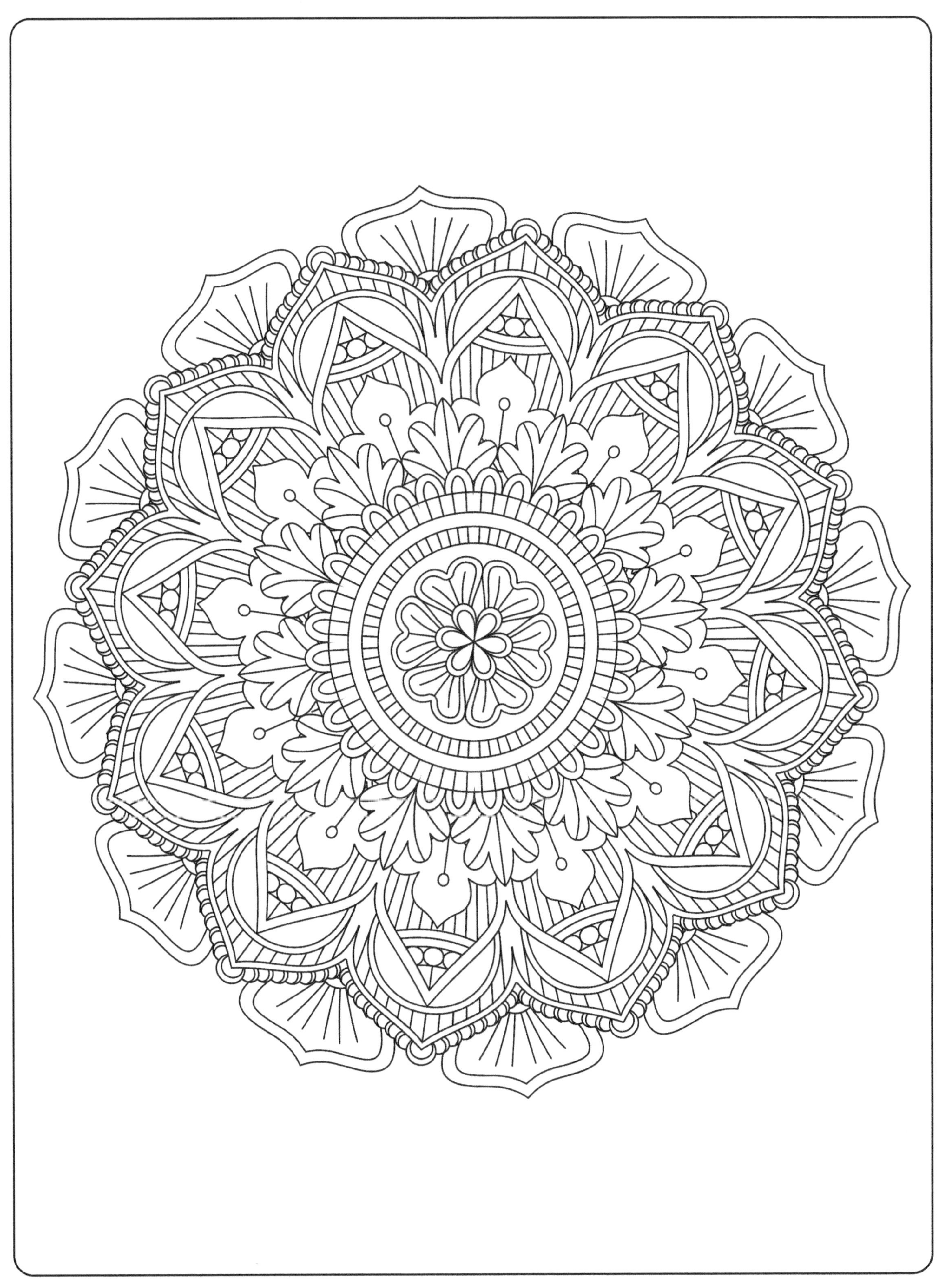

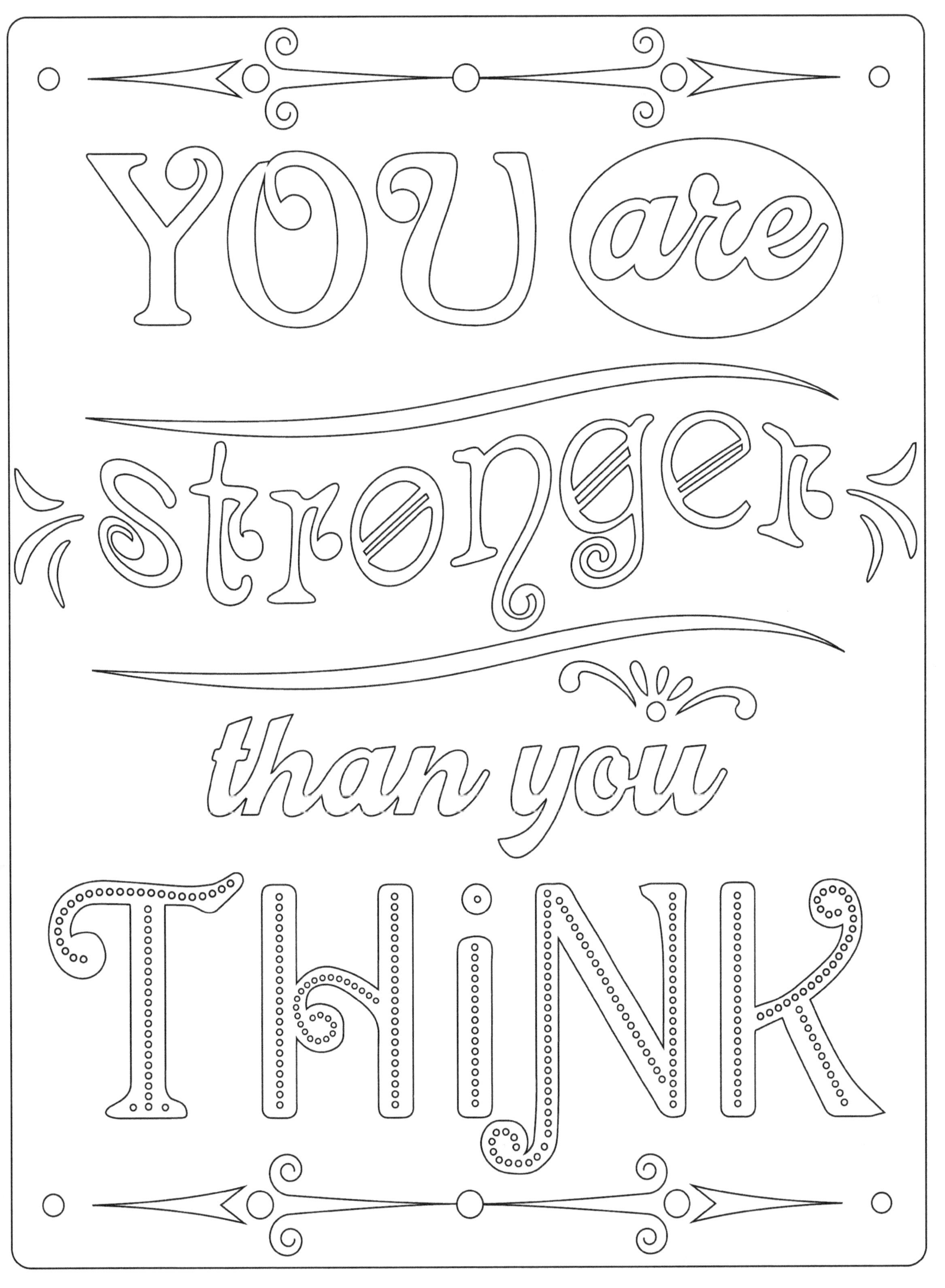

YOU are
stronger
than you
THINK

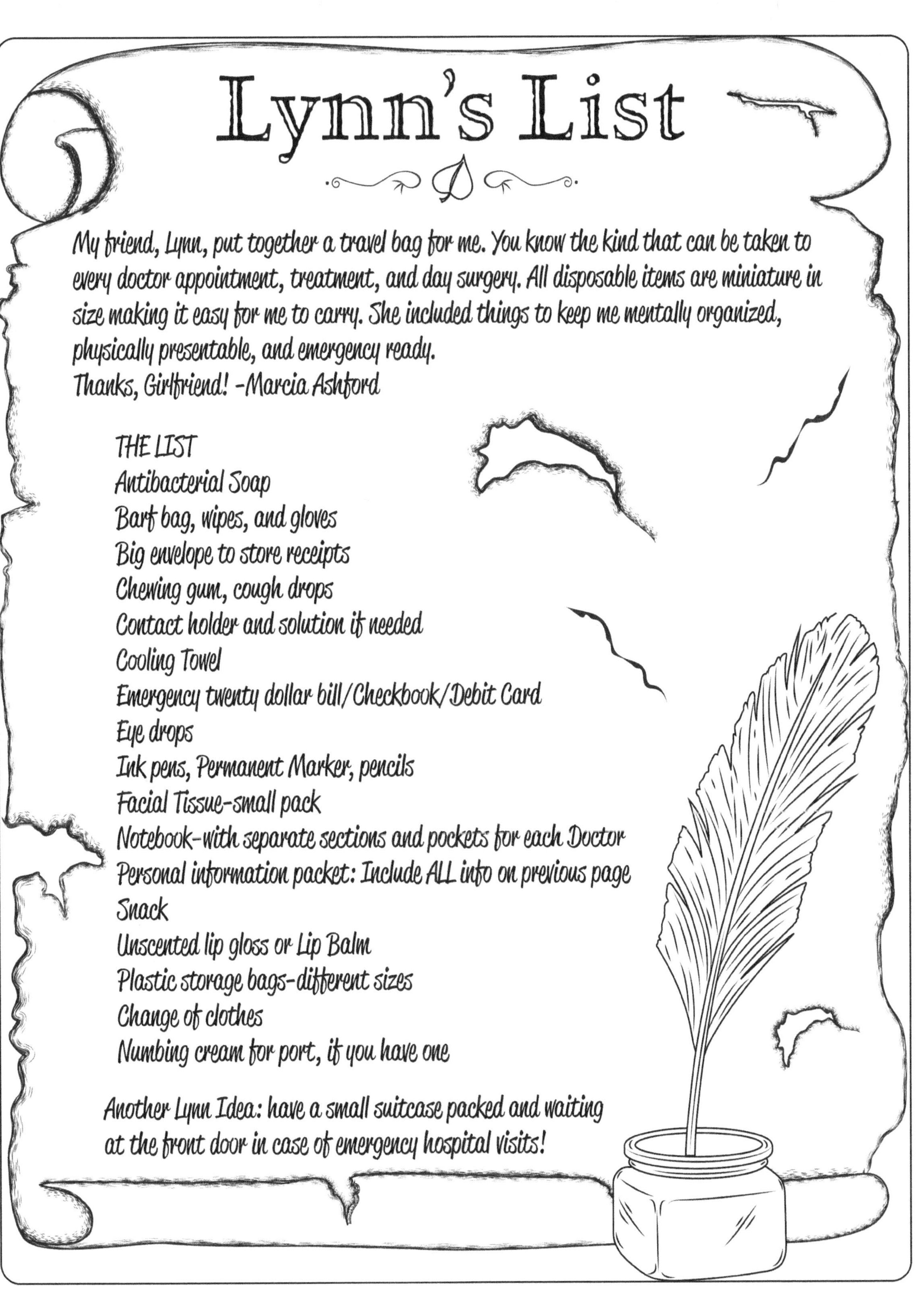

Lynn's List

My friend, Lynn, put together a travel bag for me. You know the kind that can be taken to every doctor appointment, treatment, and day surgery. All disposable items are miniature in size making it easy for me to carry. She included things to keep me mentally organized, physically presentable, and emergency ready.

Thanks, Girlfriend! –Marcia Ashford

THE LIST
Antibacterial Soap
Barf bag, wipes, and gloves
Big envelope to store receipts
Chewing gum, cough drops
Contact holder and solution if needed
Cooling Towel
Emergency twenty dollar bill/Checkbook/Debit Card
Eye drops
Ink pens, Permanent Marker, pencils
Facial Tissue-small pack
Notebook-with separate sections and pockets for each Doctor
Personal information packet: Include ALL info on previous page
Snack
Unscented lip gloss or Lip Balm
Plastic storage bags-different sizes
Change of clothes
Numbing cream for port, if you have one

Another Lynn Idea: have a small suitcase packed and waiting at the front door in case of emergency hospital visits!

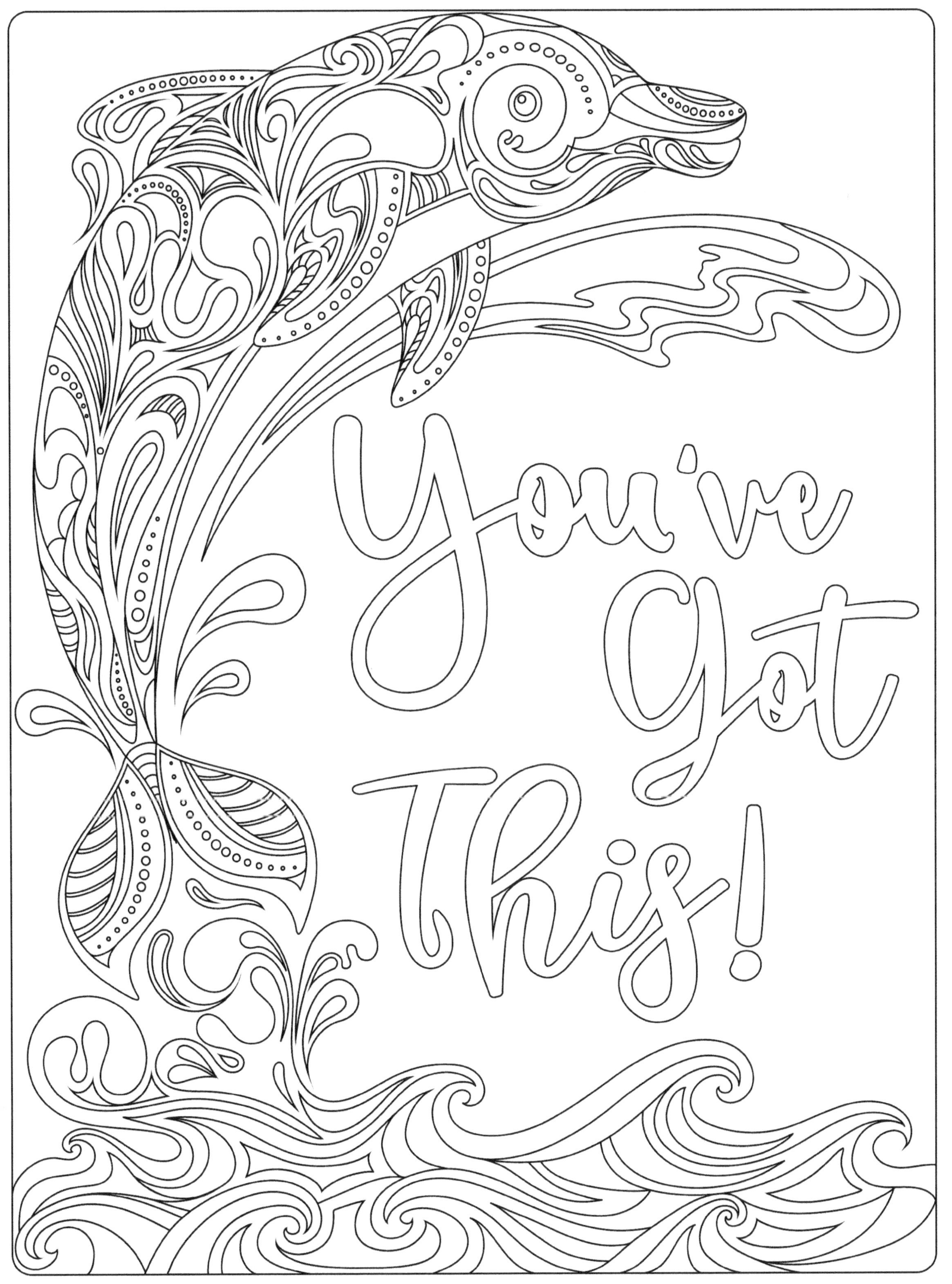

You've Got This!

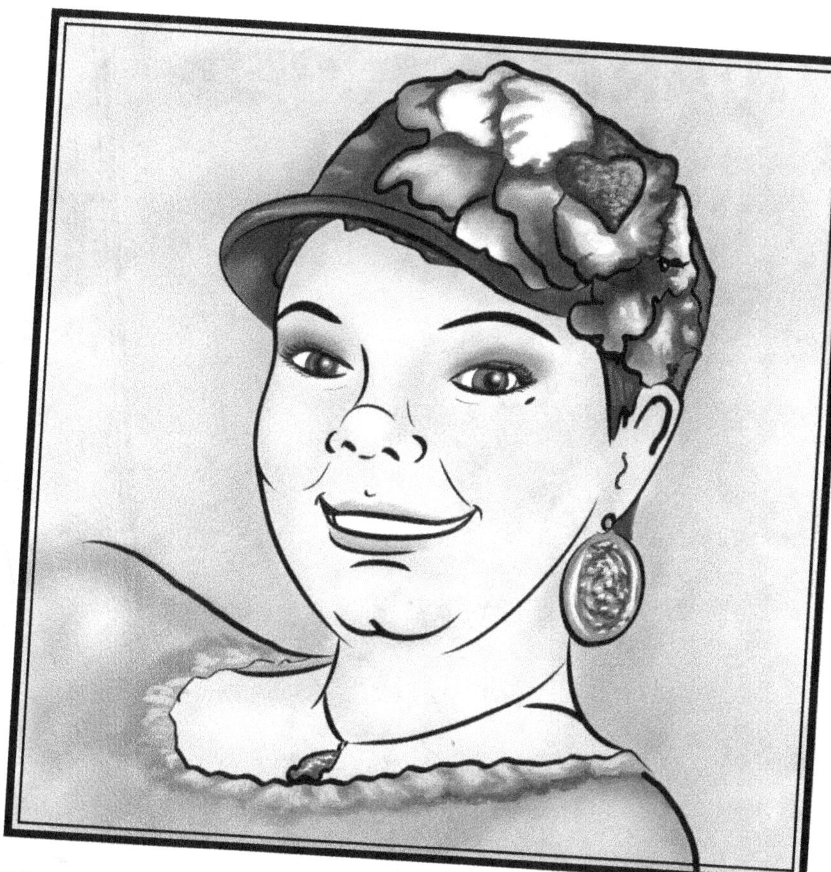

ROSLEN ROY MACK

Roslen Roy Mack is an award winning illustrator and graphic designer. She has created illustrations for over forty books and magazines. Her illustrations have been used to create and brighten many commercially manufactured products in the youth market.

Roslen is a born and raised Cajun from Lafayette, Louisiana, which means she can make a mean gumbo. Ca c'est bon! She loves drawing, cooking, playing games with the family and watching Fantasy movies. She still lives in the South with her husband, two children and their house full of pets.

She is also a Breast Cancer Survivor.

To learn more about **Roslen** visit her website at **www.dimensions-designs.com**

MARCIA MCGEE ASHFORD

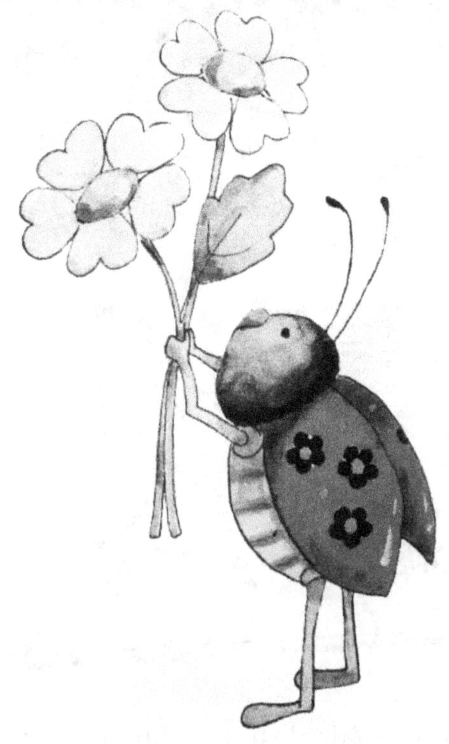

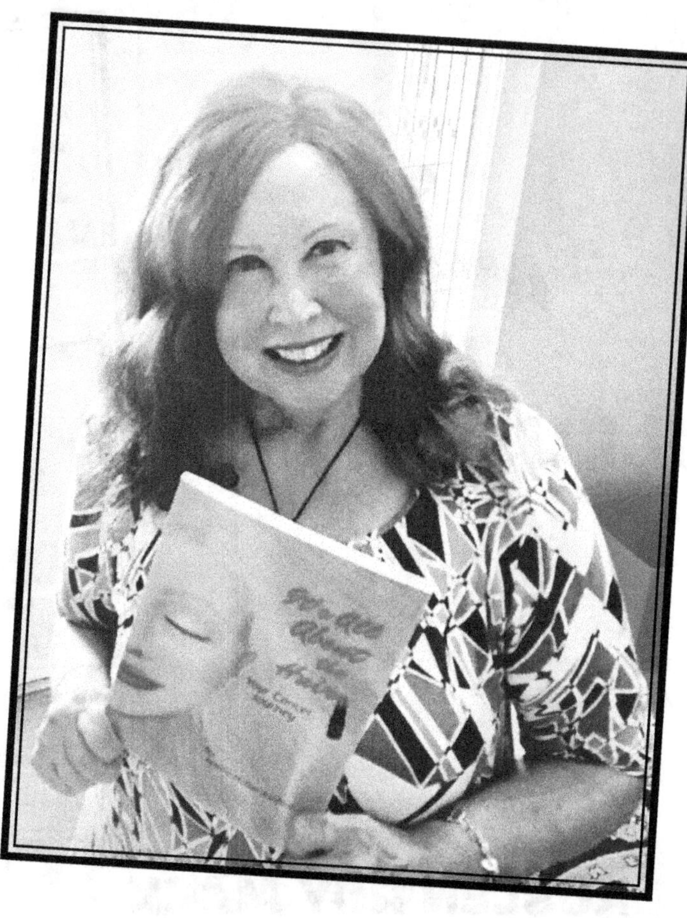

Marcia McGee Ashford, a cancer survivor, is a southern gal. She loves her family and has a passion for the beach, music, cartooning, travel, writing, "Roll Tide" football, her cocker spaniel Lexi Grace, and helping others.

She has written several books for cancer support:
It's All About the Hair, Your Cancer Journey
Life After Cancer, A Survivor's Guide
Love, Hope, Strength and Beauty, an adult coloring book for the hurting heart
A Woman's Cancer Journey will be available soon!

Her children's books:
Trudy Matoody available in English and Spanish
Trudy Matoody Coloring and Activity Book available in English and Spanish
Mommy is Sick What Do We Do?

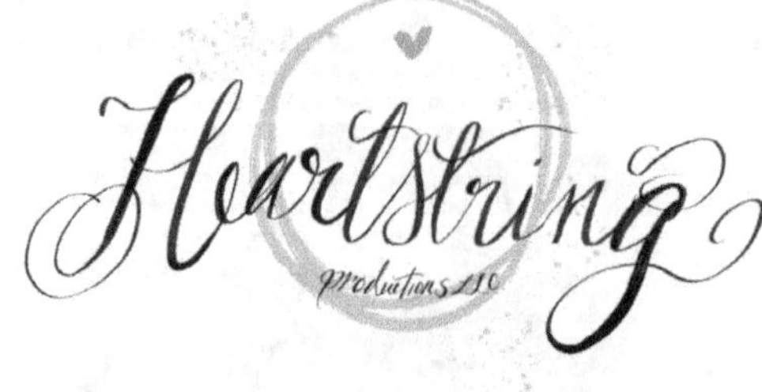

To learn more about **Marcia** visit her website at **www.heartstringproductions.com**

www.ingramcontent.com/pod-product-compliance
Lightning Source LLC
Chambersburg PA
CBHW081251250726
48654CB00012B/1574